When Stress Comes to Stay

LESA LAWSON, ND

DEDICATION

My family,
Your love, unyielding support and dependable honesty continue
to stoke the fires within me. I am but a shadow of myself
without you.

Let It Be Understood

The standard disclaimer is simply this: the information contained in this book is not intended to provide medical advice nor should it take the place of medical treatment from your own physician.

That disclaimer, however, is antithetical to my purpose. I have written to encourage people to think critically and do for themselves what no physician can do.

CONTENTS

ACKNOWLEDGMENTS

The writing of this work goes not without acknowledging my heavenly Father, my peace in the midst of stress. It is He who empowers, encourages, and emboldens me to be.

To all who lead stressful lives -namely 96 percent of mankind- holding fast to hope that you may experience true balance, honor your body, and give Stress the boot, with gusto.

LESA LAWSON, ND

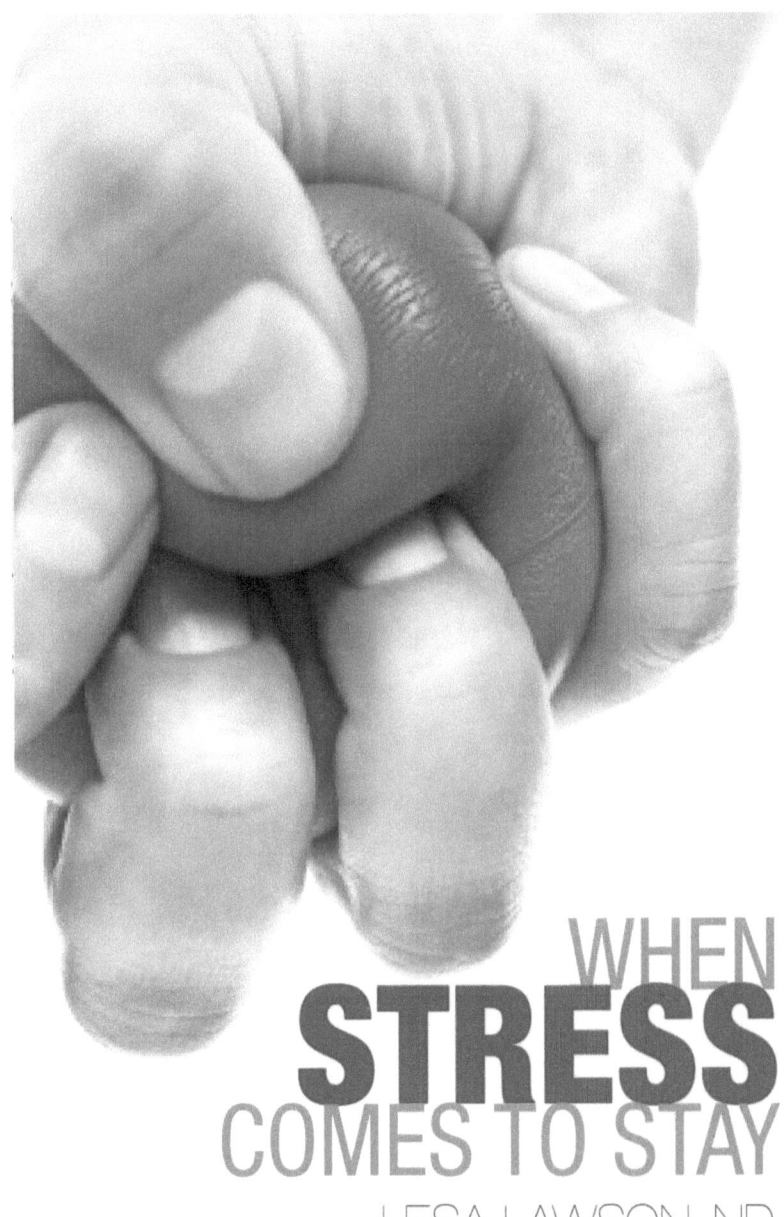

WHEN
STRESS
COMES TO STAY
LESA LAWSON, ND

INTRODUCTION

It appears in many different forms: traffic, long work hours, poor diet, fatigue, irritability, medication; and the list goes on. Regardless of how Stress appears, the end results are the same: inflammation, pain, illness, and disease. Unfortunately, many of us are unfamiliar with Stress' many disguises; as such, we are pulled relentlessly into the crashing waves, slapped about and caught helplessly in the undertow, becoming victims before we know it.

Stress is commonplace in the world but that does not mean that acceptance is our recourse. I am a firm believer in fighting for life and contending for all that ought to be ours. Stress is not our inheritance,

May this book help us become wise to Stress's devices. For conversational purposes, I have given Stress a physical body and life. May this depiction help us to see Stress for what it is in our lives: an enemy.

In disguises unveiled and others masked
sneaks Stress, the malady of man

1 THE PHILISTINES ARE UPON YOU

Despite the fact that we are of different races, hail from different places, have different last names, and coloring, there is one relative in our families who is common to us all. This relative comes to visit at the least opportune times, with lots of baggage. Tonight is no exception. Yes, without warning, without invitation, company has arrived and this promises to be an extended visit.

Stunned, you are almost trampled as adults and children barge in with mounds of baggage and chatter. They swarm around and through you, it seems, in their bid to make themselves comfortable. Already, you can feel a slight headache, as you lift some of the baggage to place… where exactly? You'll have to stack them in the hallway while you ponder that.

In the meantime, you will retrieve bedding and pillows to transform your sofas into beds of sorts, for your guests. Maybe while you're doing that, you could try to determine, delicately, of course, how long the visit will last. Well, maybe you can ask once the chatter slows.

One hour later, the thought of an early night has taken flight. You excuse yourself to hide in the bathroom, leaving your guests to finish that second 'small' snack of scrambled eggs, toast, and freshly-squeezed orange juice (no less) that you were asked to make. When you return, stubbing your toe on a suitcase that someone opened and left in the walkway, you find the meal finished and the dishes left on the table in congealing disarray. Your guests are snoring enthusiastically - right in your bed.

What to do?

Obviously, my story is fabricated but hopefully, I have stimulated your imagination. Shall I persist, then, and describe how you toss and turn on the sofa, all night, and when you finally fall asleep, your guests smack you awake, asking if you're planning to sleep all day? As they enjoy breakfast (which you made), they announce plans for the day that involve you at every turn. No consideration is given to the fact that you have a job. You're reminded, repeatedly, that you have guests.

Perhaps, for you, Stress is not at home but rather, perched on your desk at work. The latest deadline will mean late hours, insufficient rest, and rushed meals. Your class paper is overdue, or family commitments are pushed to the back burner and you're beginning to hear about them. Sound familiar?

Can you name the snarl of emotions that sweep through you? Dare I say frustration and irritation? Your jaw is clenched from holding in all that you really want to say, and that headache from last night is rearing its ugly head, promising to stay with you for the duration of the two-month visit. Two months! Will you last that long?

Over the next few days, tension hums along your shoulders, and a slight pain makes itself felt in your digestive tract. You want to run for the hills, screaming all the way. Another part of you feels a surge of something so strong that makes you want to put them right out on your doorstep, with the closed door between you, with the sofa braced against it for good measure.

What to do?

Stress holds all mankind in its sway
and adds confusion to the fray

2 MEET COUSIN STRESS

You didn't really know Stress all that well during your childhood. Quite infrequently, you met or heard about Stress, that distant relative who popped up every once in a while, and got on everybody's nerves. These days, as you've grown older, Cousin Stress seems to have taken a special liking to you. Yes, while you were 'sleeping,' Stress moved in and brought company.

Stress alone is bad enough, but with a spouse and children! Oy! Now, little Stressors are running through your life, fighting, destroying and leaving utter disaster in their wake. Okay, let's not focus on the rest of the family, just yet. That's too much to handle all at once.

Stress has awakened the "fight or flight" response in

you. "Fight or flight" is the body's biological and psychological reaction to a threat that it feels ill-equipped to handle. It is tantamount to a snarling dog running toward you and your deciding that now would be a good time to run! Sometimes, your legs take the choice from you, if you take too long to decide; then it's a case of "Feet, don't fail me now!"

When faced with a stressful situation, we either put up our fists or we run like the wind. Our decision is dependent on the way in which we view the situation and judge our chances of success. Sometimes the decision is an unconscious one. The body does not relish the prospect of being in constant battle mode; rather, it seeks methods of peace and preserving energy. In the choice of "fight or flight", we determine whether we will be victorious, and respond accordingly.

Simple decision - yes? Problem solved, Stress thwarted, move on. Unfortunately, there is a lot more to this visit than you realized. When Stress came to stay, there also came a slew of chain reactions. Stress charged a lot of purchases to your account, without your knowledge or permission, and now, it is time to pay.

Standing at the helm of our ship,
we plot and chart the course of our health or disease

3 STRESS' SNEAKY STRATEGY

You were set up, sidelined, ambushed. A childhood friend used to say, "It was a wicked and dreadful act!" Not only are you now dealing with the unfolding trauma of this visit, you're remembering the harrowing torment you endured the last time Stress came to stay.

Your heart rate hasn't seemed to slow since last night. You have no appetite, yet, conversely, you're feeling a surge of energy as you run behind the little Stressors, correcting, forestalling, and dodging disaster. That surge of energy that you are feeling is the 'fight or flight' response.

This response started in your brain the moment Stress arrived; specifically, in the area called the hypothalamus. The hypothalamus is at the base of the brain and is the father of 'fight or flight'.

Think of your situation like World War I. The hypothalamus, faced with a problem, sends for help. It sends messages to two of the body's systems, the endocrine and the autonomic nervous systems. The endocrine system contains the pituitary gland. The autonomic nervous system has a subdivision called the sympathetic nervous system containing the adrenal medulla. The adrenal medulla helps to maintain homeostasis or internal stability in the body. It keeps everything sane. The adrenal medulla joins forces with the endocrine system to handle short-term stress. We'll see whether they can handle Stress and family.

The battle is in array and more allies join the fight. The pituitary gland (from the endocrine system) and the adrenal medulla jump into the fray, bringing the liver along with them. The liver, you say? Yes, because the liver produces the glucose that is giving you the burst of whirlwind energy; the energy that will help you decide if you want to fight or flee.

War has begun! As the battle ensues, the endocrine system and the adrenal medulla begin to fall short under Stress' assault. Why? Well, you were just informed that Cousin Stress likes it here and is going to be with you for a while. Endocrine and Medulla are only equipped to fight

7

short-term stress. They can't hold the fort for long. Reinforcements will be needed. The hypothalamus will need to send a message to a super-power, the regulator of long-term stress, called the Hypothalamic Pituitary-Adrenal (HPA) system. When the HPA responds, it brings hormones along with it. Hormones mean that things are going to get interesting!

What is so interesting about hormones? Before we consider that, we probably should seek to understand what a hormone is. The Merriam-Webster dictionary defines a hormone as "a natural substance that is produced in the body and that influences the way the body grows or develops."

Hormones control and regulate the activity of certain cells or organs and are essential for every activity of life, including the processes of digestion, metabolism, growth, reproduction, and mood control.[1] Insulin, for example, is a hormone that regulates the amount of sugar in the blood (this is called glucose). Glucose is the body's main source of energy (fuel).

Why is the arrival of hormones so significant to the battle? Hormones bring control. From its arsenal, the pituitary gland discharges a substance called

---

[1] www.medicinenet.com

adrenocortisotropic hormone (ACTH) which stimulates the adrenal glands to produce a stress hormone called cortisol. Stress hormones respond to stressful or exciting situations and help return the body to a non-stressed state. Cortisol has several functions, among them releasing stored glucose from the liver.

The release of stored glucose allows the body to keep generating steady supplies of sugar to the blood, thereby producing energy. That steady supply of blood sugar helps you to cope with the Stressors.

There is one problem: while the continued over-production of blood sugar is occurring to handle prolonged stress, your immune system is suppressed. Yes, your immune protection detail stops working. Why does this happen? It's simple: your body needs to use all of its resources to handle the perceived threat that Stress brought, so your immune system is temporarily shut down to assist in the battle and deal with the problem.

Do you see the danger? If the immune system is suppressed during Stress-filled times, your defenses are down and therefore, open to attack. More on that, later; for now, let us return to the battle.

The adrenal medulla discharges the hormone, adrenaline. This hormone gets the body ready for the 'fight or flight' response. With adrenaline come changes in the body such as a decrease in digestion, increased sweating, increased pulse and blood pressure. These are responses to short-term stress.

Short-term stress does not cause ill-health. Running, workouts and other exercise could then be considered short-term stress responses, as all the symptoms listed above occur with activity. In these respects, short-term stress actually helps the body. You might wonder, then, about seemingly healthy people who collapse or die after a workout or run. Consider that there was already a problem long before the workout began.

It is long-term stress that invites ill-health.

I wear thee like a cloak; I see thee even in my dreams,
yet have I no peace concerning thee.
Clinging vine; Stress, thou art mine enemy

4 LOOK AT THIS MESS!

Short-term stress does not cause harmful effects. To use my story: if Cousin Stress were just passing through and stopped for a quick hello, you would recover, and rather quickly, too. You would shake your head, clean up, thank God that you don't have to deal with a prolonged visit, and go to bed. Since Stress will be here for a while, however, your mind has already multiplied last night's chaos by two months, added the bonus of this morning, and threw in last year's fiasco, for good measure. Your chest tightens, you're sluggish, and you feel as if you're coming down with the flu. No wonder! Your immune system has been suspended!

Here is something that many people do not know: Stress affects every area of the body. *Every area!*

Let us look at the major body systems that Stress affects.

Nervous System: brain, spinal cord, nerves

Musculoskeletal System: bones and muscles

Respiratory System: trachea, bronchi, lungs, and diaphragm

Cardiovascular System: heart and blood vessels

Endocrine System: hypothalamus, pituitary gland, thyroid, parathyroids, adrenal glands, pineal body, reproductive glands, and pancreas

Gastrointestinal System: mouth, large intestines, small intestines, stomach, gall bladder, liver and pancreas.

Reproductive System:

Male: penis, scrotum, testicles (testes), epididymis; and the accessory organs, such as the ejaculatory ducts, urethra, and prostate gland

Female: labia majora, labia minora, Bartholin's glands, and clitoris; and the internal reproductive organs: vagina, uterus (womb), ovaries, and fallopian tubes

The following diagram from the American Institute of Stress (AIS)[2] provides an explanation of the effects of Stress on the body's systems. Male or female, if Stress has you in its grasp, the repercussions are more far-reaching and can be far more devastating than we can imagine.

------

[2] http://www.stress.org/stress-effects/

Here are ways in which some **key body systems** react.

1 NERVOUS SYSTEM
When stressed — physically or psychologically — the body suddenly shifts its energy resources to fighting off the perceived threat. In what is known as the "fight or flight" response, the sympathetic nervous system signals the adrenal glands to release adrenaline and cortisol. These hormones make the heart beat faster, raise blood pressure, change the digestive process and boost glucose levels in the bloodstream. Once the crisis passes, body systems usually return to normal.

2 MUSCULOSKELETAL SYSTEM
Under stress, muscles tense up. The contraction of muscles for extended periods can trigger tension headaches, migraines and various musculoskeletal conditions.

3 RESPIRATORY SYSTEM
Stress can make you breathe harder and cause rapid breathing — or hyperventilation — which can bring on panic attacks in some people.

4 CARDIOVASCULAR SYSTEM
Acute stress — stress that is momentary, such as being stuck in traffic — causes an increase in heart rate and stronger contractions of the heart muscle. Blood vessels that direct blood to the large muscles and to the heart dilate, increasing the amount of blood pumped to these parts of the body. Repeated episodes of acute stress can cause inflammation in the coronary arteries, thought to lead to heart attack.

5 ENDOCRINE SYSTEM
Adrenal glands
When the body is stressed, the brain sends signals from the hypothalamus, causing the adrenal cortex to produce cortisol and the adrenal medulla to produce epinephrine — sometimes called the "stress hormones."

Liver
When cortisol and epinephrine are released, the liver produces more glucose, a blood sugar that would give you the energy for "fight or flight" in an emergency.

6 GASTROINTESTINAL SYSTEM
Esophagus
Stress may prompt you to eat much more or much less than you usually do. If you eat more or different foods or increase your use of tobacco or alcohol, you may experience heartburn, or acid reflux.

Stomach
Your stomach can react with "butterflies" or even nausea or pain. You may vomit if the stress is severe enough.

Bowels
Stress can affect digestion and which nutrients your intestines absorb. It can also affect how quickly food moves through your body. You may find that you have either diarrhea or constipation.

7 REPRODUCTIVE SYSTEM
In men, excess amounts of cortisol, produced under stress, can affect the normal functioning of the reproductive system. Chronic stress can impair testosterone and sperm production and cause impotence.

In women stress can cause absent or irregular menstrual cycles or more-painful periods. It can also reduce sexual desire.

With permission, from the American Institute of Stress.

Stress' Progeny

Stress's children are numerous and frustrating. Some are downright dangerous; dangerous enough to be called disorders that are emotionally and physically devastating. Look at some of their names:

- ✗ weight gain
- ✗ depression
- ✗ anxiety
- ✗ heart attack
- ✗ stroke
- ✗ hypertension
- ✗ immune system disturbances (these increase susceptibilities to infections)
- ✗ viral-linked disorders
- ✗ certain cancers
- ✗ auto-immune diseases like rheumatoid arthritis and multiple sclerosis
- ✗ rashes
- ✗ hives
- ✗ atopic dermatitis
- ✗ gastrointestinal reflux disease (GERD)
- ✗ peptic ulcer
- ✗ irritable bowel syndrome
- ✗ ulcerative colitis
- ✗ insomnia
- ✗ Parkinson's disease and other degenerative neurological disorders. [3]

---

[3] http://www.stress.org/stress-effects/#sthash.KuRHIQY8.dpuf

Yes, Stress birthed some rather destructive children and they do not belong anywhere near you. Are you now thinking that 'Fighting' is wiser than 'flight'? I agree with you. It's time to send these guests out the door and devise a plan to keep them far from you.

Stress - Innocence personified
yet roars like fire through the veins
and leaves a mark catastrophic

5 UNDERSTANDING THE SIEGE

If you are to develop a battle strategy to defeat Stress, you need to understand the full effects of the assault.

Remember this: You are at war! Your health depends on your response. Devise a strategy to undermine the threat and remove it far from you.

"Or what king would go to war against another king without first sitting down with his counselors to discuss whether his army of 10,000 could defeat the 20,000 soldiers marching against him? Luke 14:31 (NLT)

Cortisol, the Hubby

Stress has a better half: Cortisol. Cortisol is a hormone

that is secreted by the adrenal glands into the bloodstream, and helps to curtail Stress. It metabolizes glucose, regulates blood pressure, releases insulin to maintain blood sugar levels, and supports immune function and inflammatory response. Cortisol is called the stress hormone; it soothes the way after Stress wreaks havoc.

Cortisol is always present in the body but its levels vary at different times of the day. While Stress is not the only reason that cortisol is released into the bloodstream; Cortisol has still been named the "stress hormone" because its levels are decidedly higher in the bloodstream during the body's "fight or flight" response to Stress.

During short-term Stress, Cortisol is quite helpful. It helps to bring about positive effects, including lowered sensitivity to pain and sharpened memory recall. Cortisol, however, was not meant to remain at high levels in the body for long periods of time. It holds the fort, doing its part to quickly thwart Stress, thereby allowing the body to relax. Once this happens, the Cortisol level drops, as it supposed to do. Problems occur when the relaxation response is not activated in order for the body to return to normal function after the stressful event. This is where disorders and illness begin.

Society is so fast-moving and pressure-filled that our

bodies remain in stress mode for far too long. When this happens, Chronic Stress enters the picture. Chronic Stress, resulting from higher and prolonged levels of cortisol, can result in the following:

* Impaired cognitive performance (brain)
* Suppressed thyroid function
* Blood sugar imbalances such as hyperglycemia
* Decreased bone density
* Decrease in muscle tissue
* Higher blood pressure

Add to these a lowered immunity and a susceptibility to infections and illnesses, as well as a slow recovery response to inflammation which results in slow wound healing and other health consequences.

Not to be outdone, abdominal fat increases. Abdominal fat is linked to many health problems and is a far greater threat than that of fat deposited in other areas of the body. We know some of the health issues that are linked to increased abdominal fat: strokes, heart attacks, increase in "bad" blood cholesterol levels or LDL, and lower levels of "good" cholesterol (HDL).

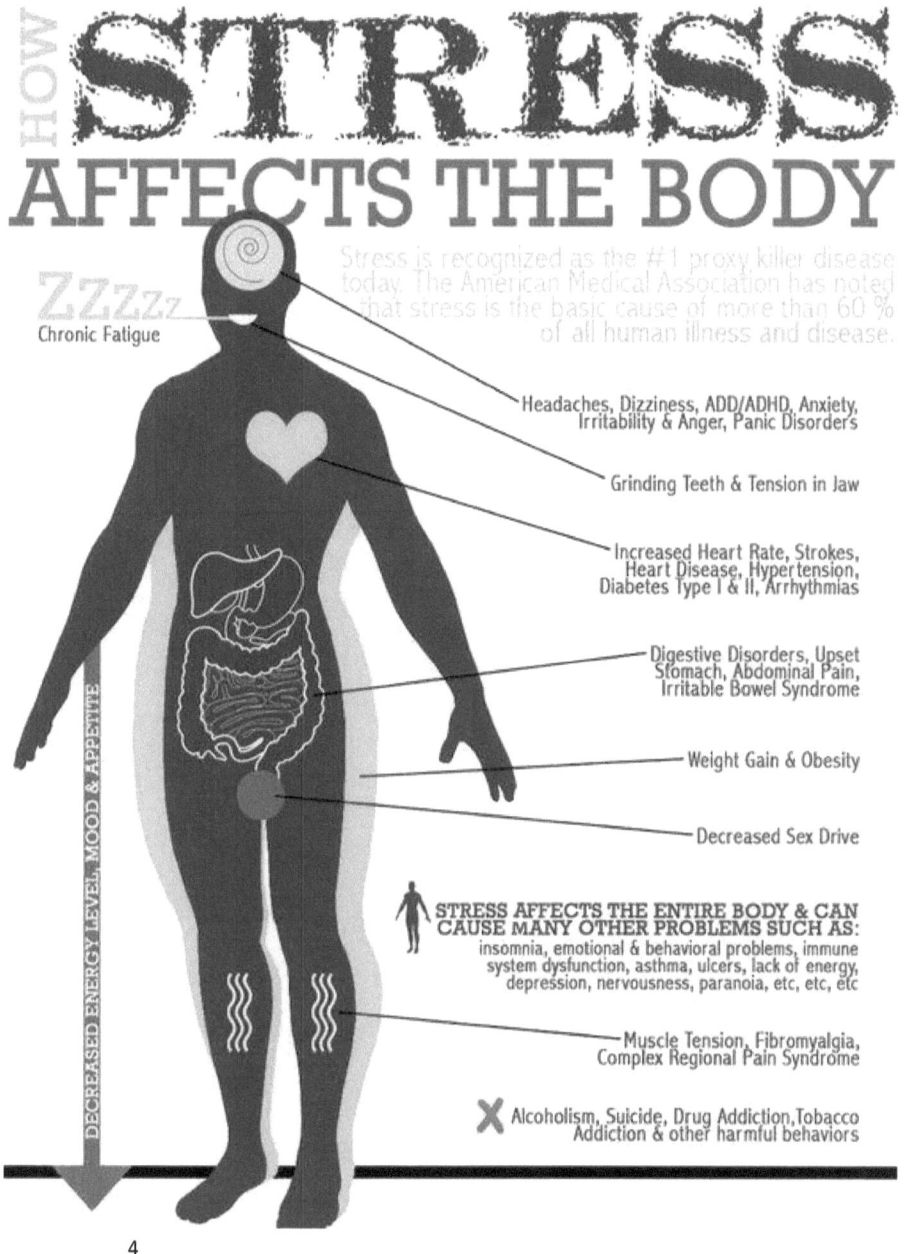

HOW STRESS AFFECTS THE BODY

Stress is recognized as the #1 proxy killer disease today. The American Medical Association has noted that stress is the basic cause of more than 60 % of all human illness and disease.

ZZZzz
Chronic Fatigue

Headaches, Dizziness, ADD/ADHD, Anxiety, Irritability & Anger, Panic Disorders

Grinding Teeth & Tension in Jaw

Increased Heart Rate, Strokes, Heart Disease, Hypertension, Diabetes Type I & II, Arrhythmias

Digestive Disorders, Upset Stomach, Abdominal Pain, Irritable Bowel Syndrome

Weight Gain & Obesity

Decreased Sex Drive

DECREASED ENERGY LEVEL, MOOD & APPETITE

STRESS AFFECTS THE ENTIRE BODY & CAN CAUSE MANY OTHER PROBLEMS SUCH AS: insomnia, emotional & behavioral problems, immune system dysfunction, asthma, ulcers, lack of energy, depression, nervousness, paranoia, etc, etc, etc

Muscle Tension, Fibromyalgia, Complex Regional Pain Syndrome

Alcoholism, Suicide, Drug Addiction, Tobacco Addiction & other harmful behaviors

4

---

[4] With permission from the Institute of HeartMath
http://empoweringwellnessnow.com/how-stress-affects-the-body/

6 STRESS AND ILLNESS

Stress's visits cause distress to the gut. This will upset the entire body, causing chain reactions that can be far-reaching. Before we proceed, let's learn more about the gut. What is the gut and where is it located?

The gut (gastrointestinal tract) is the long tube that starts at the mouth and ends at the anus (see picture, overleaf). It is an inside and outside tube, connecting and intertwining, if you will, with several organs as part of its constitution. Because it connects to so many major organs, stress from any will affect the others. Contemplate with me the reality that a pill taken for a headache may upset your stomach or that you feel fearful about a confrontation with someone and your stomach registers it. Indeed, "the digestive system is innervated through its connection with the central nervous system (CNS) and by the entric nervous system (ENS) within the wall of the gastrointestinal tract," said John B. Furness from the department of Anatomy and Neuroscience at the University of Melbourne.

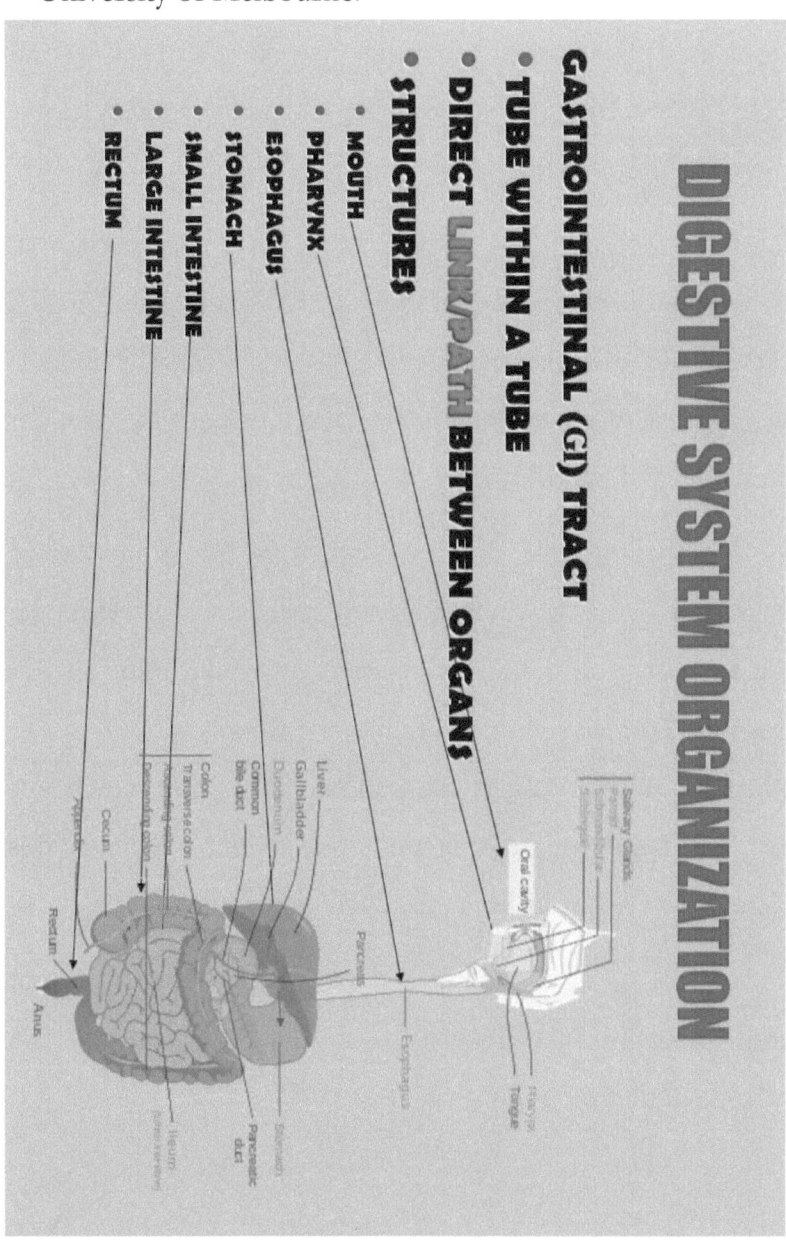

DIGESTIVE SYSTEM ORGANIZATION

- **GASTROINTESTINAL (GI) TRACT**
- **TUBE WITHIN A TUBE**
- **DIRECT LINK/PATH BETWEEN ORGANS**
- **STRUCTURES**
  - MOUTH
  - PHARYNX
  - ESOPHAGUS
  - STOMACH
  - SMALL INTESTINE
  - LARGE INTESTINE
  - RECTUM

Researchers call it the Enteric-CNS connection. Furness explains that "the ENS and CNS work in concert to control digestive function," with the CNS monitoring the state of the stomach, including its acid secretion. This explains why stress manifests itself in many digestive disorders, even though it begins as a condition of the mind. As outlined in my second book, "When Stress Comes to Stay," long-terms stress breaks down the health of the body.

Every action of the gut carries with it a huge impact on our overall health and wellness. With the brain registering all that the gut does and vice versa, consider then, that poor digestive health can affect us physically, emotionally, mentally, spiritually, and neurologically.

Most of the time, the happiness of the gut is overlooked because burgeoning symptoms seem easily assuaged with pain killers, antacids and the like. Some of us take pride in our 'cast-iron stomach' and its ability to process all the sugar, unhealthy fat, processed junk, and chemicals with which it is assaulted. Yes, the gut tolerates quite a lot. Still, even this tolerant system has its limits for ill-treatment.

Unable to filter, nullify and pacify any longer, the gut sends us signs that nothing seems to help. Congestion is one such signal that the body gives.

A visit to the doctor becomes the recourse and the doctor becomes the harbinger of disheartening diagnoses. Enter Crohn's disease, ulcerative colitis, diverticulitis, celiac disease, IBS, constipation, diarrhea, GERD, diabetes, candida, food allergies, heart disease, cancer, and even autism. Problems – yes; correctable? – definitely. The correction does, however, require something of us. Whether we choose to fulfill that requirement is exactly that – our choice.

During nerve-racking situations, digestion slows; once the problem is addressed, digestive activity increases. If the body remains in a state of continued stress, the health of the digestive system is affected. Over time, disease lurks.

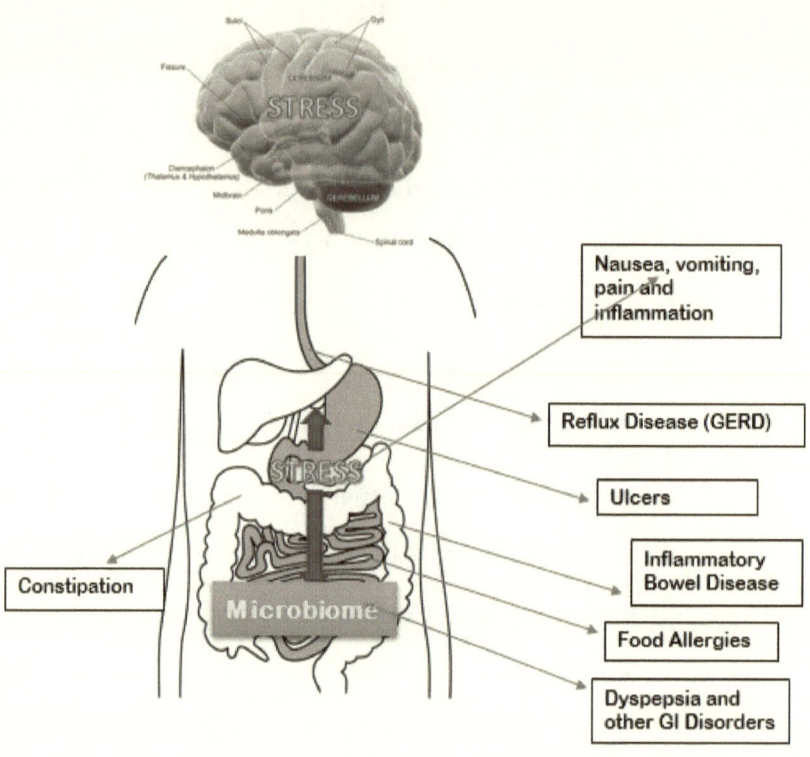

One instance of damage occurs with the prolonged production of the hormone, adrenaline, which is released during stressful situations. The continued release of adrenaline may cause ulcers.

Stress and Adrenal Fatigue

A recurrent ailment in recent years is adrenal fatigue. More and more, I see persons who are struggling with fatigue and weakness, moodiness, depression, hair loss, weight gain, and a host of adrenal fatigue symptoms, including:

* Excessive perspiration from little activity
* Lower back pain and/or knee weakness or pain, especially on the side
* Dark circles under the eyes
* Dizziness
* Muscle twitches
* Low blood sugar
* Heart palpitations
* Sensitivity to light, or difficulty seeing at night
* Cravings for salt, sweets or carbohydrates
* Low stamina for stress, and easily irritated
* Extreme mood responses after eating carbohydrates like bread, sugar, and pasta
* Chronic infections (bacterial, viral, fungal, yeast)
* Low blood pressure
* Light-headedness upon standing
* "Tired but wired" feeling; poor sleep
* Intolerance for alcohol
* Premature aging
* Dry, unhealthy skin with excess pigmentation
* Lack of libido
* Cystic breasts
* Tendency to startle easily

✖ Negative response to thyroid hormone[5]

Let us examine this debilitating condition.

Adrenal fatigue has several names: adrenal imbalance, adrenal dysfunction, exhaustion, or burnout. Regardless of the name, adrenal fatigue occurs when the adrenal glands are secreting incorrect levels of stress hormones, whether too low or too high, in relation to the amount that is actually needed by the body. This disparity often results in worrying symptoms.

When Stress occurs, your body regards the situation as an emergency, regardless of the cause. Every emergency makes demands on the adrenal glands. Your adrenals then urge your body into the "fight or flight" mode by increasing adrenaline and cortisol production. This is a survival mode response.

In its normal function, cortisol helps us to overcome Stress's challenges by converting proteins and fats into energy, maintaining our alertness, balancing electrolytes

---

[5] *"What is Adrenal Fatigue?"* www.adrenalfatigue.org

"Are You Tired and Wired? Your Proven 30 Day Plan for Overcoming Adrenal Fatigue and Feeling Fantastic Again." Marcelle Pick. 2011

(which conduct electricity), regulating heartbeat and pressure, and neutralizing inflammation. The constantly high level of cortisol is the problem because our adrenals do not know the difference between short-term and long-term Stress. The adrenals treat every situation the same, working hard whether we are stressed due to a true emergency or a bout of exercise.

When your adrenals are required to constantly respond to Stress, without rest, they eventually begin to struggle to produce cortisol, as well as key hormones like the sex hormones. This difficulty in producing hormones becomes critical as we grow older and need the full support of our adrenals to prevent extreme sex hormone fluctuations.

Adrenals and the Sex Drive

Colorful, authoritative advertising is turning us into drug-dependent love machines. When some persons begin to experience decrease in sex drive and/or sexual performance, they resort to medications which do not help in the long term. Yes, the meds might give the immediate reaction that both partners need, but over time, a reliance on the drug is created and the body has difficulty responding or functioning on its own, sexually. Soon, there is a desire for stronger doses to fix the issue.

The problem remains unfixed, though it is certainly drugged. Users must wait for a drug to take effect before they can indulge in sexual activity. Will that kill the romantic mood? I would think so! How is that true living? You are doing your body a disservice. In addition, your liver is working overtime to process the chemicals and buffer the side-effects that these drugs bring.

What causes people to resort to these drugs? Most sexual problems originate in poor diet, insufficient hydration, lack of rest, and exercise, and too much Stress. It would certainly be more beneficial to address the root cause of the problem, correct it and improve your health, so that your body can function well. Don't you believe that you are worth the time and effort?

The burden of fatigue is exhausting in itself;
that we insist on shouldering it is a wearisome paradox

7 GIVE ADRENAL FATIGUE A REST

As you are reading, you may be realizing just how stressed you really are and this may be enough to cause you anxiety. What can you do to balance your adrenals, support your body in its healing, and alleviate Stress?

Do not dismiss your symptoms. Adrenal fatigue is a condition that can, over time, become terribly debilitating. Why struggle with thyroid problems, blood pressure issues, allergies, or fatigue? If you decrease chronic Stress, learn to adjust your emotional responses to stressors, and change what, when and how you eat, you can reverse adrenal fatigue.

Examine your diet. Are you deliberately undermining your own stress response with the things that you put into your mouth?

Here's a simple assignment:

Use a notebook to create a food diary or create one on your electronic device. For about one week, do nothing to change your eating habits. Record everything that you consume, solid and liquid, even candy or cigarettes, if you smoke. Record your energy levels and overall feeling, after consuming anything. At the end of the week, look at your entries.

Do you see a pattern of any kind? Are you consuming too many fried foods or refined carbohydrates? Are there foods that cause you gastric distress? What about your sugar and salt intake; are you using too much of the sweet or salty? Are you smoking after every meal? Are you hydrating sufficiently with water?

Take note of the following contributors to adrenal fatigue:

Adrenal Stressor: Insufficient Sleep

We take rest for granted, stealing an hour from our sleep-time to make up for a shortcoming in our day. We have no set sleep patterns, so the body cannot develop a sleep habit. Do you deprive yourself five days a week, then tell yourself that you will catch up on the weekend? Have you ever proudly told someone that you "didn't sleep at all, last night", because you were online or you had a movie marathon?

Insufficient sleep causes great harm to the body. Weight gain, poor concentration, mood swings, slow reflexes, premature aging and devastating illnesses like high blood pressure, heart disease, and strokes are just some of the many problems that are couched in poor or insufficient sleep.

*Adrenal Stressor: Excess Sugar and Refined Carbohydrates

Refined carbohydrates (carbs) are foods that have been processed and are no longer in their natural state. They have been depleted of their life force and stripped of the natural minerals and vitamins with which they were created.

Refined carbs. digest very quickly, which can lead to surges in blood sugar levels. After the sugar spike, energy levels tend to drop. When blood sugar levels drop, and so quickly, some people experience weakness, shakiness, headaches, fatigue or sleepiness. The adrenals then rush to produce stress hormones to raise the blood sugar again. As blood sugar rises and falls, over and over, it puts strains on the adrenals, resulting in low blood sugar or reactive hypoglycemia. This may also lead to food cravings, which may then lead to weight gain.

The reason that we experience "the shakes" and some of the other reactions is that the body cannot metabolize or utilize pure, refined starch and carbohydrates unless their previously removed proteins, vitamins and minerals are present. Because these carbohydrates and starches are refined, thereby providing little if any nutritive value, when we consume them, there occurs incomplete carbohydrate metabolism. Toxic metabolites are formed because of the incomplete carbohydrate metabolism.

These toxic metabolites interfere with the respiration of the body's cells, according to Dr. William Coda Martin in his 1957 explanation of why sugar is a poison. In time, Dr. Martin, stated, some of the cells die, interfering with the function of a part of the body, and is the beginning of degenerative disease. [6]

Daily intakes of refined sugar not only rob your body of minerals but can also change the body's pH and increase acidity. The body, in its effort to metabolize sugar, will extract minerals and vitamins (especially B vitamins) from your joints

[6] *The Dangers of Refined Sugar*, Dr. William Coda Martin, The Michigan Organic News. 1957

and tissues. This results in deficiencies and so. Most sugars, flours and rice are refined and unnatural.

Given all the different types of advertising, some persons cannot readily identify refined carbohydrates. Here's a quick definition ditty that will help:

Refined Defined

If it into the oven went
or frying pan and oil it knew,
then comes to you in box or bag,
Refined it is and not for you

Liquids refreshing and so sweet
have added sugars, all refined.
Sodas and energy drinks; sweet tea
will, in time, make you lose your mind

White flours, pasta, corn syrup, too,
and all the pies and cakes they make
Biscuits and waffles, breads and buns
are sure to cause your joints to ache

Now, last, not least, are all the names
of sugars, they all end in 'ose'
Galactose, sucrose, dextrose – strange
All of them rhyme with comatose

~Lesa Lawson, ND

Interpretation:

~Snack Foods~

Most snacks have long shelf lives because they have been stripped of the nutrients that make them living foods. The grains used to make the flour are stripped of the beneficial bran and germ. Dead foods are of no value to the body. These products have lots of salt and sodium (these two are not the same). Refined snacks include biscuits, crackers, cookies, candies, chips, pretzels and most snack bars.

~White Breads and Pasta~

Foods made with white or all-purpose flour are refined carbohydrates (carbs). If you look at the ingredients of these refined foods, the first or second ingredient is "enriched" flour. This means that the nutrients were stripped from the grain during the refining process, then, synthetic imitations of nutrients were added afterwards. The body isn't fooled; it does not digest synthetic ingredients well. Remember the toxic metabolites from incomplete carbohydrate metabolism.

Refined carbs are digestible because the fiber has been removed. When these carbs are eaten, they are broken down carbs into sugar. Therefore, in addition to the sugar that is

~Other Refined Foods~

White rice, instant oatmeal, pancake mixes, and most desserts; white sugar (table sugar), brown sugar, pancake syrup, honey, agave, corn syrup, and high fructose corn syrup are also refined.

Adrenal Stressor: Caffeine and other Stimulants

Stimulants are substances that raise the levels of physiological or nervous activity in the body, and increase activity in the brain. While they can temporarily elevate alertness and mood, stimulants (among them caffeine, alcohol, energy drinks, cigarettes, diet pills and powders) activate the release of extra stress hormones, which can exhaust the adrenal system.

Caffeine, in addition to being a stimulant, is also a diuretic, meaning that it increases urine production and can contribute to dehydration. If you drink a lot of coffee, hopefully, you're also drinking lots of pure water.

Alcohol, even in small quantities, inhibits the absorption of the B vitamins, namely thiamine (B_1), riboflavin (B_2) niacin (B_3), biotin (B_7), folic acid (B_9), and cyanocobalamin (B12).

The B vitamins help in the manufacture of red blood cells and deficiency often results in anemia, causing weakness and tiredness. Vitamin B-12 is vital in the production of brain chemicals that help with mood and other key brain functions. Low levels of B-12 and B-6 have been linked to depression. Regular drinking of alcohol decreases vitamin B12 absorption from the gastrointestinal tract.

Adrenal Stressor: Dehydration

Yes, you knew that this one was coming. Dehydration affects every cell in the body. When your body is dehydrated, it undergoes major stress. Your body will let you know by signaling thirst but if you decide to feed it sweet drinks or energy drinks, it will soon show its dissatisfaction through joint pains, muscle cramps, constipation, sour stomach, sunken eyes, headaches, weariness and drowsiness. My mom always says that there is no cure for sleep but sleep; the same is true for water. Water does for the body what no other liquid can do.

Adrenal Stressor: Food Sensitivities and Allergies

Food allergies and sensitivities are quite common. They are immunological responses to substances that we consume, be they spices, additives to foods, certain ingredients or the foods, themselves. Many of us who had no such condition in our childhood or younger years, are now reacting to certain foods. Some people are allergic to nightshade foods (tomatoes, eggplant, peppers, and white or Irish potatoes). There are also wheat, dairy, gluten, soy, sugar and yeast, corn, and food dye allergies.

Eating foods, repeatedly, that cause you to have an allergic reaction can strain adrenal function, causing inflammation and fatigue in the adrenal glands.

Adrenal Stressor: Poor Bowel Movements and Habits

In the busy scramble of life, bowel movements are pushed to the back of the line. Every time we do this, we are training our bodies to forego a natural function. The body does not like it but since we are in charge, it has no choice. After a time of doing this, it barely registers on our consciousness that there is no regularity; or that the stool is hard or that we have to strain or the stool is dark and putrid.

By the time we are forced to pay attention, it is because the body raises a clamor through heartburn, stomach aches or other issues, constipation or spots of blood in the stool. Constipation leads to other problems and those problems don't always swim blissfully away in the laxative that we quickly seize at the pharmacy. In fact, many times, laxatives compound the problem. One result of constipation and constant laxative use is adrenal strain.

*Adrenal Stressor: Digestive Concerns

Many women and yes, men, have a proliferation of Candida (yeast) in their gut, along with excessive bad bacteria from poor dietary habits and undigested food. The standard diet of white flour, white sugar, white rice, with sugary drinks and other non-foods is also a major contributor. This combination leads to gut inflammation and chronic infections. Eventually, the rest of the body begins to suffer because no part of the body works in isolation. All of these conditions, of course, place strain on the adrenals.

Adrenal Stressor: Inflammation

Inflammation invades every part of the body, including the brain. In addition to Candida, constant, chronic stress, poor diet, dehydration, and over-acidity are some of the causes of inflammation in the body. When there is inflammation in the brain, there is the tendency towards forgetfulness, low concentration, brain fog, brain pain, and low alertness.

Adrenal Stressor: Untreated Autoimmune Disease

Autoimmune disease is the end result of the immune system attacking the body's own tissues or organs, rather than defending it. Some organs that are affected by autoimmune diseases are the pancreas (Diabetes Mellitus type 1), the thyroid gland (Hashimoto's hypothyroidism), and the nervous system (Multiple Sclerosis).

Adrenal Stressor: Excessive Exercise

I can see the smiles on some faces, so let me hasten to clarify. Exercise is essential. It oxygenates the brain and blood, prevents the heart from becoming sluggish, strengthens the bones and is simply vital. Over-exercising, on the other hand, can tax the adrenals and cause you to feel so tired that you can hardly function. If you notice that your workouts leave you feeling strangely lethargic, you might need to reduce the intensity or frequency.

Let us now examine ways to support our adrenals, improve energy, and sustain our body during its inherent healing process.

The body will heal if we treat it well
and if we don't, there'll be hell to pay

8 FOOD FOR THOUGHT AND ACTION

We have discussed how certain foods cause blood sugar to surge and further stress the adrenals. Adopting a low-glycemic, whole foods program is essential, as low-glycemic foods do not generally have a significant effect on blood sugar. Include healthy fats, protein, and fiber in your diet (see the Glycemic Index chart for examples).

The Glycemic Index (GI) measures the way in which carbohydrate-containing food raises blood sugar. Foods with a rating of 56 and above will raise the blood sugar more than those at 55 and below. Low GI diets have been linked to reduced risk of type 2 diabetes, cardiovascular disease, stroke, depression, and chronic kidney disease, formation of gall stones, formation of uterine fibroids, and cancers of the breast, colon, prostate, and pancreas."[10]

High and Low Glycemic Foods

The following information concerning the Glycemic Index was taken from http://www.the-gi-diet.org/lowgifoods.

Study the table below to plan more healthy meals. The number listed next to each food is its glycemic rating or index. This value was obtained by monitoring a person's blood sugar after he ate the food. The value can vary slightly from person to person and from one type or brand of food or another. The GI rating of Special-K cereal showed significantly different findings in tests in the US and Australia. This, according to the study, most likely resulted from different ingredients in each location. Despite this variation, the index is a guide as to the foods to eat and avoid. Note the GI index range:

---

[10] The World's Healthiest Foods.
http://www.whfoods.com/genpage.php?tname=faq&dbid=32

GI Index Ranges
Low GI = 55 or less, Medium GI = 56 – 69, High GI = 70 or more

Breakfast Cereal

Low GI

All-bran (UK/Aus)	30
All-bran (US)	50
Oat bran	50
Rolled Oats	51
Special K (UK/Aus)	54
Natural Muesli	40
Porridge	58

Medium GI

Bran Buds	58
Mini Wheats	58
Nutrigrain	66
Shredded Wheat	67
Porridge Oats	63
Special K (US)	69

High GI

Cornflakes	80
Sultana Bran	73
Branflakes	74
Coco Pops	77
Puffed Wheat	80
Oats in Honey Bake	77
Team	82
Total	76
Cheerios	74
Rice Krispies	82
Weetabix	74

Staples

Low GI

Wheat Pasta Shapes	54
New Potatoes	54

Bread

Low GI

Soya and Linseed	36
Wholegrain Pumpernickel	46
Heavy Mixed Grain	45
Whole Wheat	49
Sourdough Rye	48
Sourdough Wheat	54

Medium GI

Croissant	67
Hamburger bun	61
Pita, white	57
Wholemeal Rye	62

High GI

White bread	71
Bagel	72
French Baguette	95

Snacks and Sweet Foods

Low GI

Slim-Fast meal replacement	27
Snickers Bar (high fat)	41
Nut & Seed Muesli Bar	49
Sponge Cake	46
Nutella	33
Milk Chocolate	42
Hummus	6
Peanuts	13

Vegetables

Low GI

Frozen Green Peas	39
Frozen Sweet Corn	47
Raw Carrots	16
Boiled Carrots	41
Eggplant/Aubergine	15
Broccoli	10
Cauliflower	15
Cabbage	10
Mushrooms	10
Tomatoes	15
Chilies	10
Lettuce	10
Green Beans	15
Red Peppers	10
Onions	10

Medium GI

Beetroot	64

High GI

Pumpkin	75
Parsnips	97

Fruits

Low GI

Cherries	22
Plums	24
Grapefruits	25
Peaches	28
Peaches, canned in natural juice	30
Apples	34
Pears	41
Dried Apricots	32
Grapes	43
Coconuts	45
Coconut Milk	41
Kiwi Fruits	47

Meat Ravioli	39	Walnuts	15	Oranges	40
Spaghetti	32	Cashew Nuts	25	Strawberries	40
Tortellini (Cheese)	50	Nuts and Raisins	21	Prunes	29
Egg Fettuccini	32	Jam	51		
Brown Rice	50	Corn Chips	42	**Medium GI**	
Buckwheat	51			Mangoes	60
White long grain rice	50	Oatmeal Crackers	55	Sultanas	56
Pearled Barley	22			Bananas	58
Yam	35	**Medium GI**		Raisins	64
Sweet Potatoes	48	Ryvita	63	Papayas	60
Instant Noodles	47	Digestives	59	Figs	61
Wheat Tortilla	30	Blueberry muffin	59	Pineapples	66
Medium GI		Honey	58		
Basmati Rice	58	**High GI**		**High GI**	
Couscous	61	Pretzels	83	Watermelons	80
Cornmeal	68	Water Crackers	78	Dates	103
Taco Shells	68	Rice cakes	87	*Dairy*	
Gnocchi	68	Puffed Crispbread	81	**Low GI**	
Canned Potatoes	61	Donuts	76	Whole milk	31
Chinese (Rice) Vermicelli	58	Scones	92	Skimmed milk	32
Baked Potatoes	60	Maple flavored syrup	68	Chocolate milk	42
Wild Rice	57			Sweetened yoghurt	33
		Legumes (Beans)		Artificially Sweetened Yoghurt	23
High GI		**Low GI**		Custard	35
Instant White Rice	87	Kidney Beans (canned)	52	Soy Milk	44
Glutinous Rice	86	Butter Beans	36		
Short Grain White Rice	83	Chick Peas	42	**Medium GI**	
Tapioca	70	Haricot/Navy Beans	31	Ice-cream	62
Fresh Mashed Potatoes	73	Lentils, Red	21		
French Fries	75	Lentils, Green	30		
Instant Mashed Potatoes	80	Pinto Beans	45		
		Black-eyed Beans	50		
		Yellow Split Peas	32		
		Medium GI			
		Beans in Tomato Sauce	56		

Food Allergy Testing

Your primary care doctor can perform allergy testing to determine which foods provide negative reactions. Sometimes, the tests provide a negative reading, when people are, in fact, allergic to a particular food. Here is a simple way to test and double-check at home: perform an elimination/re-introduction test and note your results. You can then discuss your results with your doctor and he/she can then help you plan a course of action.

How to Do the Elimination Test

Find your food diary that you created and look at the foods that are problematic. Avoid those foods for about seven days or until the symptoms that you experienced have disappeared completely.

During this time of avoidance, your body is being cleansed of the problem food. Once there is no longer a reaction at all, reintroduce each food, one at a time. And wait for four days, between introductions. If you eat more than one of the problem foods at the same time, you won't be sure which is the cause of the allergy. Eat one food at least twice in one day, then do not eat it again for at least four days. Note your internal and external reactions. If you have a reaction, it is possible that you are allergic to that food. If there is no reaction, then re-introduce the next food item.

Please be patient and prepare yourself for the fact that the elimination test may take a few months, for some persons, depending on the severity of the food reaction and, also, the time that it takes for all symptoms to abate. You can adopt the four-day rotation for problem foods, to help reduce your symptoms. If the rotation diet does not bring relief for a certain food, then you should consider eliminating that food, altogether. It took me a long time to accept that I needed to eliminate dairy and wheat but I finally got the message. Those two foods must be second cousins to Stress because they sure brought Stress to me!

Meals: Timing is Everything

When we go for long periods of time without food, our blood sugar drops, causing a stress reaction. Our adrenal glands must then work hard to release extra amounts of he hormones, cortisol and adrenaline, to try to maintain the body's normal functioning.

The body always needs energy, even at rest, though obviously, it doesn't need as much when we are asleep. Cortisol works to balance blood sugar levels in-between meals and even during sleep; therefore, we need to keep our cortisol levels regulated by eating timely, healthy meals. Eating, however, too frequently, is also counter-productive. Eat meals that provide nutrients and fiber to keep you full and satisfied.

Cortisol levels follow our natural circadian rhythm. The circadian rhythm is the body's internal clock; the rhythmic activity cycle that occurs in a person or thing within a 24-hour period. For humans, the circadian rhythm begins to rise at about 6 a.m., peaks at about 8 a.m., and then, throughout the day naturally rises and falls as needed. It tapers off at night, and reaches its lowest levels while we are sleeping.

Eating large meals earlier in the day will help to support cortisol levels, and a smaller, lighter meal at the end of the day will help maintain hormonal balance.

I am not a proponent of six or more small meals per day. Having nutritionally beneficial and satisfying meals that contain a variety of food groups is vital. Vegetables and fiber, with good protein, whether animal or vegetable, and some *unrefined* carbohydrate, will keep you satisfied and prevent continued snacking. This is not to say that we cannot ever have a snack. We just need to make sure that our meals are nutritionally dense enough to keep blood sugar stable and adrenal levels as normal as possible.

Give your organs a rest with some kind of intermittent fasting during the day. Don't eat all day; eat your meals within a certain window of time [an eight-hour window is good] and then stop.

Do not consume too much animal protein but do have protein at every meal. This should, always be animal protein. Choose grass-fed, hormone-free, organic meats, if you eat beef, lamb, mutton or goat. If buying chicken, look for free-range, organic poultry. The same applies to eggs. Fish should always be wild-caught, never farm-raised. Buy fish and meat that do not have color added to them.

Plant sources of protein include lentils, hemp and chia seeds, spinach, avocado and others that are listed below.

Breakfast and the Adrenals

Some people skip breakfast because they do not feel hungry. This is a mistake. Breakfast does not have to be large but it should be eaten and should be wholesome and nutritious. If you consistently do not feel hungry in the morning, you could have some adrenal fatigue which can cause a decrease in liver function and suppress normal morning hunger. This must be addressed.

Include good protein in your breakfast. Eggs, especially egg yolks are helpful to the adrenals because they are high in amino acids and B vitamins. There are also many sources of vegetarian protein that are easy on the digestive system and are great to include in the first meal of the day. Here are some sources:

Quinoa and Other Whole Grains

Quinoa has the highest protein content of all grains. It also contains all of the essential amino acids, thereby making it a "complete protein". One cup of cooked quinoa contains 18 grams of protein, as well as nine grams of fiber. Brown rice and millet provide healthy protein, as well. Consider having the latter two in the middle of the day or afternoon. Soak brown rice to remove some of the phytic acid and enable faster cooking. Don't forget to pour off the water that you used to soak the rice. Rinse and then cook with clean water.

Consider eating sprouted grains. They are easy to digest and are high in nutrients.

Beans, Lentils and Legumes

Beans, lentils, kidney beans, split peas, chickpeas, Indian dhal, split pea soup and chickpea hummus are all protein-rich. Of course, there are others kinds of legumes. To avoid bloating or gas, wash and soak beans overnight, then discard that soaking water and add fresh water before cooking. Adding a piece of fresh ginger or the sea vegetable, kombu to the cooking of beans and peas will also help to decrease flatulence.

Nuts, Seeds and Nut Butters

Nuts like cashews, almonds, and walnuts and seeds such as chia, hemp, sesame, and sunflower seeds are protein-rich. Sprouted nuts and seeds are more easily digested and are higher in nutrients than their counterparts. Use chia, flax, and hemp seeds in smoothies. Ground chia seeds contain healthy omega 3s. Try almond, cashew nut butters or sunflower butters. Avoid peanuts and peanut butter; they are not easily digested and cause more digestive issues than people realize.

The oils of choice are coconut and olive and the cold-pressed varieties are the most beneficial. Healthy fats and oils can help to stabilize blood sugar levels. Use them for cooking or in salads or for oil pulling.

Vegetables that Support the Adrenals

Adrenal powerhouse vegetables include beet, celery, Swiss chard, kelp, kale, red peppers, spinach, sprouts, butternut and yellow squash, olives (green and black), and zucchini. Add cultured (fermented) vegetables like sauerkraut, pickles, fermented beets, and kimchi to your diet to obtain live, active probiotic cultures. These fermented foods help to replenish good bacteria in the gut, thereby helping the adrenals, too.

The good bacteria (lactobacilli) that are responsible for the fermentation (like those in sauerkraut, kimchee, yogurt or other cultured foods) will repopulate in your intestinal tract and help your body manufacture its own B vitamins.

Consider making your own fermented vegetables for a constant supply. Culturing your own vegetables is quite easy. Make sure to use Himalayan or Celtic sea salt if you choose to make your own (See web links for sauerkraut and Kimchi recipes at the end of this section).

Sea vegetables like dulse, nori, wakame, kombu, and hijiki are excellent for the adrenals and may be added to your fermented recipes.

A Note on Fermented Foods

If you have digestive problems, they are difficult to heal completely, if the gut health balance is not improved. You need to re-establish the balance between the good, beneficial bacteria and the disease-causing bacteria that exist in your gut. Fermented foods will help. They are rich in lactic acid–producing bacteria. Fermented foods help to balance the production of stomach acid, increasing gastric juices that help digestion, when needed, or protecting the lining of the stomach and intestines, if there is too much acid. Either way, digestive distress is eased.

Fermented foods help to relieve constipation, acts as a digestive aid, strengthens the microbiome, thereby strengthening the immune system, and is even helpful to those with diabetes, as these pre-digested carbohydrates take pressure off the pancreas. Have a serving of pickled vegetables with at least two of your daily meals. Try making some; it is easy to do. I have provided a simple sauerkraut recipe on the next page. Give it a try.

Sauerkraut

(Makes 2 quarts)

- 2 quart glass jar
- 2 head cabbage (red or green), shredded chopped (leave 2 whole leaves to cover the mixture)
- 3 carrots, cut into strips
- 2 turnips kohlrabi or turnips, white radish, broccoli stems, beets, etc. cut into thin slices (optional)
- 10g salt per 450g of veggies (about 2½ teaspoons)

Directions

- Sprinkle the cabbage and vegetables with salt in a large bowl.

- Pound the cabbage with a wooden pounder for 10-12 minutes or massage until the cabbage releases its juices.

- Pack mixture into the jar, tightly, until the juices cover the veggies (cover with the whole leaves and add a weight to keep the veggies submerged in the liquid). Set the jar in a container because juices may run over during the fermentation process.

- Cover jar and store in a pantry for 10 days to one month – tasting every few days to ensure the vegetables are souring nicely. Make sure to uncover at least once daily.

TIP: If the top starts to brown, stir the sauerkraut and pack down the veggies below the juices.

Note from Dr. David Williams, Medical Researcher:

It's normal for white spots or a white film to form on the surface of the liquid covering the sauerkraut. It's a form of yeast called kahm. Although it's totally harmless, it can impart a bad taste to the cabbage so simply remove it, gently, with a spoon before removing any of the sauerkraut.

1. **An Easy Salt-Free Sauerkraut Recipe**
   http://bit.ly/1s1Ta7Q

2. **Homemade Sauerkraut in a Mason Jar**
   http://bit.ly/1d6k7Q9

3. **Salt-free Kimchi**
   http://bit.ly/2dEgb7e

4. **Regular Kimchi**
   http://bit.ly/2ehyu0u

Salt and the Adrenals

Salt can help adrenal fatigue. **Please note**: use Celtic sea salt or Himalayan sea salt. Include it in your cooking (in small doses, of course) or in your green juices or smoothies. If energy levels are low, consider adding a pinch to a ¼ teaspoon of either salt to pure or purified water upon waking.

Hydration and the Adrenals

Drink lots of pure water throughout the day. Your joints, brain, in fact, your entire body needs it! How much water should you drink? First, calculate the amount of water that your body needs. Sedentary tasks, desks jobs and low-energy activities may require just the minimum water requirement (see method, below), that which your body needs to function. If you are exercising, hiking or doing high energy, strenuous jobs, you will need more than the minimum requirement. Don't gulp! Rather, drink slowly and allow your body to put the water to use.

Method: Divide your body weight in half. If, for example, you weigh 140 pounds, drink 70 ounces of water, per day, if you are within the sedentary or lower energy category. For high energy jobs and activities, increase your intake.

Liquids for Stress Reduction

Make teas out of ginseng (Panax), valerian, chamomile and passionflower herbs. Fresh, green juices and smoothies of kale, spinach, carrot, and lemon or other combinations are also quite beneficial.

Oils for the Adrenals and Stress Reduction

Essential oils are extremely helpful to the endocrine system. Oils that are pure and of therapeutic grade assure safe internal use. If you are unsure as to the therapeutic grade of the oil, use it externally or in a diffuser, only. When using externally, use a carrier oil. Carrier oils, like coconut, almond or safflower, help with absorption, while protecting the skin's delicate tissues.

The pure essential oils produced by **Nature's Sunshine** and **dōTERRA®**[11] are of therapeutic grade (may be used internally) as well as applied topically and used in a diffuser. Utilize as many natural methods as possible to support your body on its way to recovery. Essential oils constitute one such method.

Where Should You Apply Essential Oils?

The most common areas on which to apply oils for adrenal and hormonal support are the back of the neck, the reflex points on the ankles, lower back, thyroid, liver, kidneys and gland areas, the center line of the body, and along the sides of 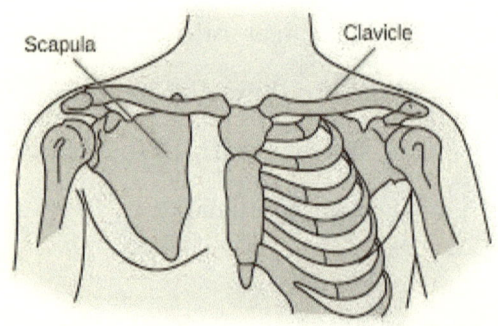 the spine, and area of the clavicle (collarbone region).

---

[11] To order from Nature's Sunshine or dōTERRA®, see the last page.

Some helpful essential oils that support the adrenals include:

Peppermint	**Lavender**
Chamomile	**Clove Bud**
Basil	**Vanilla**
Rose	**Lemon Balm**
Rosemary	**Nutmeg**
Frankincense (Boswelia)	

Note:

Some oils are gentle and do not require dilution before topical application. Oils such as **Lavender** and **Serenity** fall within this category. Some essential oils are stronger (e.g. **Cinnamon bark** or **Oregano**), and should be diluted with coconut oil prior to being applied to the skin.

Always dilute the oils when using on children, unless the oils are being applied to the bottoms of their feet. Consider the same strategy with sensitive individuals and the elderly.

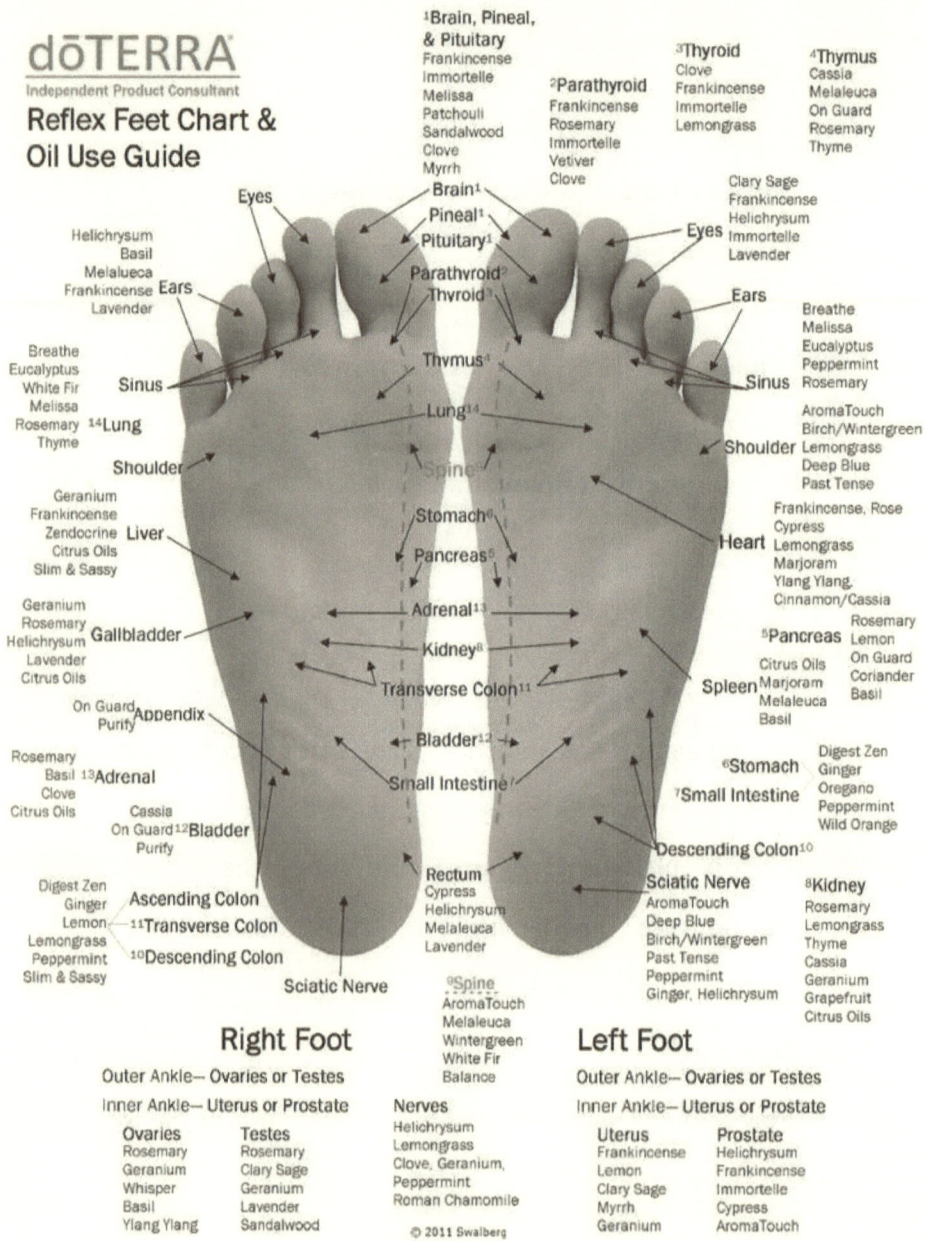

dōTERRA

Independent Product Consultant

Reflex Feet Chart & Oil Use Guide

¹Brain, Pineal, & Pituitary
Frankincense
Immortelle
Melissa
Patchouli
Sandalwood
Clove
Myrrh

²Parathyroid
Frankincense
Rosemary
Immortelle
Vetiver
Clove

³Thyroid
Clove
Frankincense
Immortelle
Lemongrass

⁴Thymus
Cassia
Melaleuca
On Guard
Rosemary
Thyme

Eyes
Helichrysum
Basil
Melalueca
Frankincense
Lavender
Ears

Brain¹
Pineal¹
Pituitary¹
Parathyroid²
Thyroid³

Eyes
Clary Sage
Frankincense
Helichrysum
Immortelle
Lavender

Ears

Breathe
Eucalyptus
White Fir
Melissa
Rosemary
Thyme
Sinus
¹⁴Lung

Thymus⁴

Lung¹⁴

Spine

Sinus

Breathe
Melissa
Eucalyptus
Peppermint
Rosemary

Shoulder

Shoulder

AromaTouch
Birch/Wintergreen
Lemongrass
Deep Blue
Past Tense

Geranium
Frankincense
Zendocrine Liver
Citrus Oils
Slim & Sassy

Stomach⁶

Pancreas⁵

Heart

Frankincense, Rose
Cypress
Lemongrass
Marjoram
Ylang Ylang
Cinnamon/Cassia

Geranium
Rosemary
Helichrysum Gallbladder
Lavender
Citrus Oils

Adrenal¹³

Kidney⁸

Transverse Colon¹¹

⁵Pancreas

Spleen

Rosemary
Lemon
On Guard
Coriander
Basil

Citrus Oils
Marjoram
Melaleuca
Basil

On Guard
Purity Appendix

Bladder¹²

Rosemary
Basil ¹³Adrenal
Clove
Citrus Oils

Small Intestine⁷

⁶Stomach

⁷Small Intestine

Digest Zen
Ginger
Oregano
Peppermint
Wild Orange

Cassia
On Guard¹²Bladder
Purity

Descending Colon¹⁰

Digest Zen
Ginger
Lemon ¹¹Transverse Colon
Lemongrass
Peppermint
Slim & Sassy ¹⁰Descending Colon

Ascending Colon

Rectum
Cypress
Helichrysum
Melaleuca
Lavender

Sciatic Nerve
AromaTouch
Deep Blue
Birch/Wintergreen
Past Tense
Peppermint
Ginger, Helichrysum

⁸Kidney
Rosemary
Lemongrass
Thyme
Cassia
Geranium
Grapefruit
Citrus Oils

Sciatic Nerve

⁹Spine
AromaTouch
Melaleuca
Wintergreen
White Fir
Balance

Right Foot

Outer Ankle— Ovaries or Testes

Inner Ankle— Uterus or Prostate

Ovaries	Testes
Rosemary	Rosemary
Geranium	Clary Sage
Whisper	Geranium
Basil	Lavender
Ylang Ylang	Sandalwood

Nerves
Helichrysum
Lemongrass
Clove, Geranium,
Peppermint
Roman Chamomile

© 2011 Swalberg

Left Foot

Outer Ankle— Ovaries or Testes

Inner Ankle— Uterus or Prostate

Uterus	Prostate
Frankincense	Helichrysum
Lemon	Frankincense
Clary Sage	Immortelle
Myrrh	Cypress
Geranium	AromaTouch

Aromatools.com

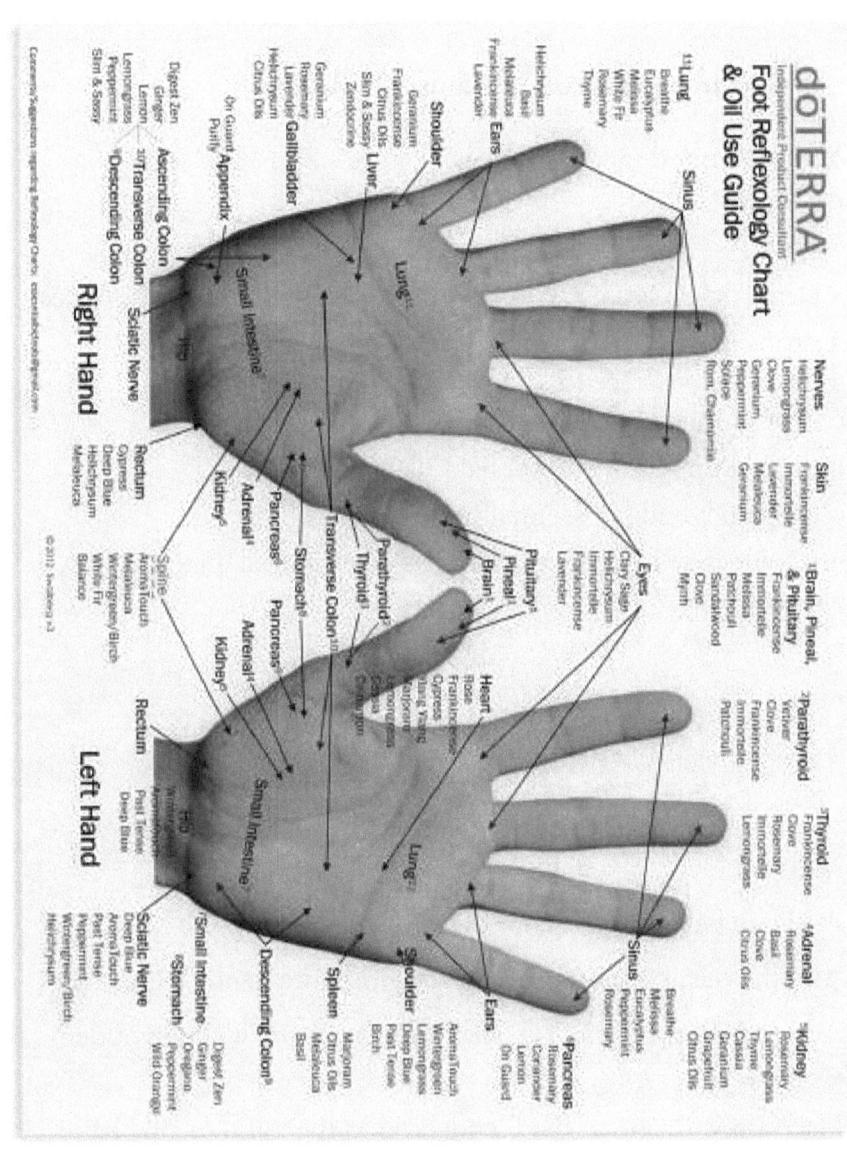

Aromatools.com

Recipes and Protocols

Adrenal Support Essential Oil Recipe

You will need (available from Nature's Sunshine and dōTERRA®):

1 clean, dry Glass jar with cover (able to hold least 4-6 ounces)

4 drops Rosemary Essential Oil

4 drops Clove Essential Oil

6 drops Clary Sage Essential Oil

4 drops Peppermint Essential Oil

6 drops Lavender Essential Oil

4-6 ounces of a carrier oil, such as coconut oil, jojoba oil or almond oil.

Optional:

4 drops Basil Essential Oil

Method:

Add one half of the carrier oil to the glass jar.

Add the oils, one at a time, shaking mixture gently to blend.

Add remaining carrier oil, shake gently or stir with a wooden spoon.

Place a few drops of the blended oil in the palm of one hand.

Rub the combination on your adrenals, which are located on your lower back, just above your kidneys.

Adrenal Support Protocols - dōTERRA®

[All dōTERRA® supplements contain essential oils]

Support: Use **PB Assist** to provide your body with live bacteria and pure essential oils. Apply **Zendocrine oil blend**, topically, over the area of the adrenals. The oils in the **Zendocrine oil blend** work to gently cleanse and filter the liver and kidneys.

Elimination: Add fresh lemon or lime juice and a drop or two of **lemon oil** to room-temperature water, first thing in the morning, to get the digestive system moving. Limes and lemons do wonders for the digestive system, and also help with alkalinity.

Anxiety and Mood Support: **Citrus Bliss, Lavender,** and **Serenity** help to boost the mood. Apply topically or use aromatically in a diffuser.

Hormone Support: Use 2 drops of **Frankincense oil** under the tongue, morning and night. Use **Geranium oil**, topically, over the kidneys. Use 2 drops of **Balance oil blend** on the soles of the feet, morning and night.

Remember that any oil that is too strong for you can be taken in capsules. **dōTERRA®** supplies empty capsules for your convenience.

Since stress affects us on many levels, here are some other oil combinations that provide support:

Relief of Fatigue: Ginger, Peppermint, White Fir, Life Long Vitality Pack (LLV). Inhale Peppermint and White Fir, use on the temples or use in a diffuser. Ginger, applied topically to the areas of the liver and adrenal glands, is also quite helpful.

Fatigue Treatment #2: Take 6 drops of Slim & Sassy Oil Blend and 3 drops each of Peppermint Oil and Wild Orange Oil in a capsule daily. Rub 2-3 drops of Citrus Bliss Oil Blends on the bottoms of feet each morning. Take the **Life Long Vitality Pack**, daily.

Impotence: Clove, **Clary Sage**, Ginger, **Sandalwood**, Ylang Ylang

Libido Support: **Sandalwood**, Ylang Ylang, Ginger, **Peppermint**, Elevation, **Clary Sage**

Low Blood Sugar: Cinnamon, Clove, Thyme, Slim and Sassy Blend

Migraines: Past Tense, Peppermint**, Frankincense**

Mood swings: **LLV, Clary Calm,** Bergamot, **Clary Sage**, Fennel, **Geranium,** Lavender, Lemon, **Peppermint**, Rosemary, **Sandalwood**, Blue Spruce, Ylang Ylang

PMS: **Clary Calm,** Bergamot, **Clary Sage**, Fennel**, Geranium**, Grapefruit, Lavender, Roman Chamomile

Prostate support: Helichrysum, **Immortelle**

Descriptions of the Powerhouse Oils for Adrenal Support:

The oils that are in bold, above, provide great support for the body. Here is some information about them, including application steps:

Geranium and Frankincense – help to balance the entire body.

Frankincense also supports the endocrine system. Place 2 or 3 drops under the tongue, morning and night.

Zendocrine - Supports healthy cleansing and filtering functions of the liver, kidneys, colon, lungs, and skin.

Clary Calm (specific blend to balance hormones); also manages PMS symptoms - Apply to bottoms of feet, back of the neck, the temples and/or inhale the aroma.

Balance – benefits all systems, bringing calm while increasing focus. Wonderful for hormonal support.

Whisper – Oil for many hormonal conditions; it helps both men and women.

Sandalwood: Supports the hormones. Supports testosterone levels. Mix with **Frankincense** to balance the thyroid and endocrine system. Helps to support the hypothalamus.

Melissa – for fatigue, depression, and menstrual support. Melissa also kills virus before it enters the cell.

Balance and Geranium – hypothyroid and adrenals – rub on lymph nodes on the neck and inside of the wrists for one week; then rotate with lemongrass, myrrh, peppermint and clove for one week. Alternate until a feeling of balance returns.

Past Tense – for joint pain, inflammation, chronic pain, and arthritis. This oil is good for headaches and migraines resulting from hormone imbalance.

The **Life Long Vitality Pack** contains balanced supplements and oils to boost energy levels. Ginger, Peppermint, and White Fir used individually or applied together, are restorative.

Supplements for Adrenal Health

I love Ashwagandha! It is such a powerful herb that supports the immune system. Along with Ashwagandha, there are other herbs, minerals and vitamins that support the adrenals and help the body to heal after extended periods of stress.

B vitamins are exceedingly helpful, along with vitamins C and E. Magnesium, calcium, zinc, manganese, selenium, and iodine also help to support the body during times of stress.

Food sources of B vitamins include whole, unprocessed foods, turkey, tuna and liver, legumes (pulses or beans), whole grains, potatoes, bananas, chili peppers, tempeh, nutritional yeast, brewer's yeast, and blackstrap molasses.

The B12 vitamins are not available from plant products, making B12 deficiency a valid concern for vegans. The elderly may need to supplement their intake of B vitamins due to problems with absorption, and athletes may need to supplement their intake because of increased needs for energy production.

Use the B vitamins with Ashwagandha and Siberian ginseng. You can also try Astragalus, Licorice or Schisandra roots. Work with a botanical expert or herbalist for the best combination.

Your adrenal glands are energy regulators. Treat them well and they will return the favor.

Adrenal Support Protocols – Nature's Sunshine

Support: Two good supplements for balancing adrenals are **Adrenal Support** and **Nervous Fatigue Formula**. Persons who have chronic anxiety and nervousness and especially those who struggle with post-traumatic stress disorder are most times in need of **Adrenal Support**. Sometimes, they may need even stronger adrenal glandular support.

Other Supplements

Lobelia - highly valued for anxiety, **Lobelia** relaxes all the muscles of the body, helping to relieve spasms, cramps, and tension. It is fairly strong and is best used for acute cases of anxiety or the occasional need to relax. While relaxing the muscles, *Lobelia* slows and strengthens the heartbeat, expands the respiratory passageways, and calms breathing.

STRESS-J - a milder nervine formula more suited to daily use for prevention of anxiety and stress, this formula is recommended for stress, nervousness, anxiety, addictions, hyperactivity, chest pain and other nervous disorders.

Licorice Root - **Licorice** sustains the kidneys, spleen, liver, stomach, and pancreas, helps to stabilize blood sugar levels, and is useful in helping individuals who use caffeine and other substances that tend to vacillate the adrenals. For blood sugar problems, stress, or weak adrenals. take two capsules with breakfast, two capsules with lunch, and, if fatigued in the afternoon, two capsules with a midafternoon snack.

Nutri-Calm- Another combination for stress is **Nutri-Calm**. This vitamin/mineral supplement helps those who are highly excitable and nervous and is also used to help hyperactivity, nervous disorders, schizophrenia, stress, depression, sleeplessness, and drug withdrawal.

Take one tablet three times a day to calm the nerves.

Nervous Fatigue Formula is for those persons who struggle with emotional problems, exhaustion, insomnia, memory problems, nervous disorders, restlessness, disturbing dreams, and low sex drive. Take three capsules with a meal three times a day.

AnxiousLess – This formula is used by persons who struggle with overwhelming feelings of nervousness, apprehension, irritability, insecurity, and anxiety generally during job interviews, public speaking, flights, first dates, major deadlines, final exams, etc.

Stress Protocol (Nature's Sunshine)

Nervous System Pack
Nutri-Calm
Nerve Control
Nerve Eight
Kava

These supplements work together, synergistically, to calm the body, while refreshing and nourishing the nerves. Remember that every time we deal with long-term stress, the body loses a lot of minerals and vitamins in the attack.

Run for the Prize

After food and supplements, take a look at your physical activity. If you are doing too little exercise or none at all, your adrenals can also be affected. Hold the running and intense workouts for the moment. Exercise increases cortisol levels, so perform lighter activities while trying to heal adrenal fatigue.

To keep cortisol levels as balanced as possible, perform the more heavy exercise in the morning or early afternoon when cortisol is higher. Reserve your stretching, walking and light exercises for the evening. Try to walk for at least 20-30 minutes, each day. Walk slowly, at first, then increase your pace and time as you feel better.

Constipation Remedies

Wholesome foods, pure water, exercise, and natural remedies for adrenal recovery will all help to overcome constipation. Olive oil and coconut oil are most helpful. Taking one teaspoon, in the morning, on an empty stomach, then increasing, after a few weeks to one tablespoon will aid lubrication of the colon. You can also take one teaspoon before bed. If the taste is an issue, try following it with fresh lemon juice in a glass of water. Note: This water must *not* be cold.

The following essential oils from doTERRA will also help: GX Assist (digestive enzymes, PB Assist (probiotic), and Zendocrine Capsules. The following help with digestion: Digest Zen (oils or softgels), Black Pepper, Fennel, and Peppermint.

Colon hydrotherapy is also a most effective and excellent way to evacuate the contents of the bowel. If you are experiencing constipation or continuous diarrhea, consider doing some colon hydrotherapy sessions. If you have never had one, consider doing at least three. The first two should be done with one day in-between and the last one about three days later. Make sure to hydrate quite well at least 24 hours before your session. Your colon hydrotherapist will advise you on how to prepare.

Sleep is *Not* Over-rated!

We all need rest. Stress and poor lifestyle habits can affect serotonin, melatonin and other hormones that aid sleep. Try to get at least eight hours of sleep and make an effort to go to bed at the same time, every night, before or by 10:00 p.m. Not only does this train the body but there are added benefits that occur between 11 p.m. and 2 a.m.

The body cycles through sleep stages. For most, our deepest sleep occurs between 11 p.m. and 2 a.m. During this stage, the body repairs and regenerates tissues, builds bone and muscle, and strengthens the immune system. The body's hormonal system also cleanses between 11pm and 1am. There are many processes that occur while you are sleeping. Healing is a major one, so go to bed and go to bed on time. You will also slow your aging if you get sufficient rest and at the right times.

Deep Breathing

Practice deep breathing throughout the day. This will help to oxygenate the brain and bring calmness and alertness. Here's a simple method that I have adapted from Dr. John Douillard. Make sure that you are sitting (but not driving) or lying down because you might become lightheaded the first few times that you do it.

Breathing Exercise

1. Read instructions, first, and then close your eyes

2. Keep your mouth closed and breathe in and out through your nose for 30 seconds. Breathe deeply and exhale forcefully, as if trying to expel something from your nose.

3. When you have mentally counted to 30, hold your breath for 15-20 seconds and think of something calming. Keep your eyes closed the entire time. The exercise will last about one minute and you can repeat it several times throughout the day.

Oxygen intake can also be increased by taking a brisk, 10-minute walk and breathing only through your nose for the duration. This will boost oxygen levels and serotonin. You will be pleasantly surprised at how energized and alert you will feel. In addition, proper hydration with pure, alkaline water, eating an alkaline diet, and consuming healthy fatty acids will also aid oxygenation. If you keep at it, Stress will begin to see the writing on the wall.

Wisdom is the cloak that experience wears
to clothe the nakedness of utter folly

9 WHEN STRESS MOVED IN WITH ME

There I was, twenty-nine years old, with enough problems to donate my body to science for years of research. I had been given several diagnoses, some with names so long that I could have used them to form my own alphabet. Fatigue had become my first name, with nausea vying avidly for the spot. I was achy, constantly having colds, the flu or some other malady, and having daily headaches and pains up the wazoo (though as to exactly where that was, I'm still deciding); and the list went on until it looped.

My life became a frustrating cycle of hospital visits, referrals to specialists who poked, prodded, and said 'hmm' all the time, repeated tests and consultations, and constantly administered medications, some of which were still in the testing stages. I became a fascination, a subject of furrowed brow study; in short, a guinea pig. Doctors pegged me with the following diagnoses:

- Arthritis
- Gastrointestinal Reflux Disease (GERD)
- H-Pylori infection
- Migraines
- Possible Multiple Sclerosis
- Food allergies
- Nickel allergy
- Severe immunodeficiency and lowered immune function
- paralysis from the waist downwards due to a drug reaction (I dragged myself around on my belly for three weeks)

With all that we have discussed, I'm sure you can read the signs by now but at that time, I had no clue. What I did have was a host of medications to match every proffered diagnosis. I kept my doctors puzzled, even after four years of testing and treatments because their diagnoses and eventual surgery did not correct, slow, nay, even skim the root of the problem. This was new to them. It was new to me, too.

Growing up in the country, in Jamaica, had given me lots

of health advantages. Our childhood food was devoid of chemicals; we ate from local, well-known farmers. Maybe the most that we had to fear was seafood, although toxic dumping into Caribbean waters, while possible, was unheard of, then.

We grew quite healthily and were rarely ill; then came school lunches. I remembered that I liked the milk that came in little pink and white boxes at school (the milk was pink too); however, the milk did not like me. For me, cow's milk and diarrhea were spelt the same way, so I started to avoid milk.

Fast forward to the late 1990s: I was living in the USA and had begun to have stomach pain and headaches. The apartment in which I lived had a bad case of mold but no one knew about it, then (my landlady was always ill and her daughter had become ill and died in that house; still all of that was for later discovery).

My diet was not that great; I had veered from the healthy eating habits of my childhood. Initially, the stomach pain could be ignored but as time went by, it became a nagging companion. I noticed that it became worse with certain foods and avoided them; still ice-cream, pizza, and Kentucky Fried Chicken were on the menu. I had not yet made the connection.

My life was rather hectic in Brooklyn, New York. Church and job were fairly close to home. I had very little "me" time. My day-to-day existence was as follows:

- Monday through Friday, I awakened at 4:00 a.m. and got ready for 5:00 a.m. prayer at my church. I walked to church (15 brisk minutes) and stayed until 7:00 a.m.

- I walked to the bus stop (15 minutes), then rode the bus for an additional 25 minutes.

- Work lasted from 8:00 a.m. to 4:00 p.m., after which, I went to school by bus or taxi.

- I attended classes from 4:30 p.m. until 7:30 p.m., then walked or took a taxi to choir rehearsal or some other gathering. Those lasted until about 9:00 p.m. on Tuesdays, Wednesdays and Fridays.

- I either walked or got a ride home, then would do homework or study before preparing for bed. When my job moved to New Jersey, I added an additional 2 hours of travel to my day.

- Saturdays brought prayer at 6:30 a.m. and other activities that lasted until 9:30 a.m. Laundry and other activities took the rest of the day. Sunday was an all-day excursion. I was a member of the praise team and choir; I was also a Sunday

School teacher, youth leader, and assistant director for both youth and adult choirs. Rehearsals before and after church. Yikes!

Stress had a stranglehold on my life but I didn't even think of it and neither did my doctors. Add to my schedule, my less-than-stellar eating habits, and the mold that, unknown to me, lived within the walls of my apartment. I was surely headed for disaster.

Thus began a round of doctors, diagnoses, and drugs, among them *Aciphex*, *Cimetadine*, *Nexium* (acid blockers), *Celebrex* (anti-inflammatory), *Prednisone* (immunosuppressant steroid), and *Cipro* (anti-bacterial drug, also used in the treatment of inhaled Anthrax).

Over a period of three years, I became so ill that I regurgitated everything that I tried to eat. At one point, the only thing that would stay in my stomach was Schweppes Ginger Ale. I couldn't even tolerate water but now I know that the water in our pipes, in the States, is horribly impure and highly acidic. Ironically, although I was not eating, I was not losing weight; I weighed 160 lbs., further perplexing my doctors, since I was consuming only ginger ale and medications.

One day, after careful examination by a new specialist, he

told me that my organs were shutting down. I didn't really hear much of anything after that. Instead, I focused on the roaring in my ears and the sudden rush of warmth radiating from the top of my head. The words 'shutting down' meant imminent death, preceded by horrible pain, in my mind. I envisioned myself unable to control my lower faculties and being left in a hospice to bemoan my last few days, punctuated by pitiful drops of drool that I could not even wipe.

It did not help that the doctors did not know what was wrong with me. On top of all the drugs they prescribed which made me more ill, they performed an EMG (huge needles!) MRIs, an endoscopy, and CT Scans. All this led to major surgery but the problems persisted and I was later told that the surgery wasn't really necessary. That day, hearing those words from the specialist brought me to the river's edge; I took no more drugs. My liver could take no more, anyway. Instead, I took my health in hand, keeping my own food diary and incorporating much of what I am sharing with you.

Now, wiser, healed and trained, I'm able to help you who are heading in the direction that I was or who are already there.

10 MOVING INTO THE NEW

Now that you have been armed with knowledge, you may be able to start decreasing your stress right away. Recognizing the ill-effects within yourself is the first step to fixing poor lifestyle habits. Some of you will struggle and that struggle may lead to excess cortisol production.

Not everyone can handle stress on his/her own. For me, some changes were easy and quick and some took longer than I liked. I had to remind myself that it takes time to heal. Now, I am reminding you. It took years to develop the consequences of unhealthy habits; equally, it will take time to renew your body. Be patient. Get help. Call me. Schedule a consultation. My contact information is on the last pages of this book.

You are definitely worth the time it takes to be well. If

you haven't given it thought, look in the mirror and don't avoid those knowing eyes.

Are they tired? Are there bags or circles under them? Have they been there for a long time? Are the whites of your eyes beginning to yellow? Are there spots and dots on the white parts of the eyes?

Are you well?

That person inside you, screaming to be released from the prison of pain, procrastination and passivity, is up for parole.

What will you do?

Eight Steps to Thwart Stress

Your body is a brilliant creation, yet easy to maintain. Use these steps to help bring clarity and reduce stress.

Try to have...

One mental health day per week (or at least one hour) Relax...

Two servings of fruit, daily (try a new fruit, each week).

Three days of exercise (at least). Walk up and down your stairs (10-30 minutes); walk outside or through the mall.

Four servings of vegetables, daily (at least). Add fatty acids.

Five minutes of reflection, daily. Start an "I am thankful" journal.

Six minutes of prayer (at least). Connecting to your heavenly Father is life-changing!

Seven morning meals (Not seven meals a day but rather, have breakfast, everyday)

Eight glasses of water, daily (at least; regardless of what you hear). Get at least eight hours of sleep, too!

ON A PERSONAL NOTE

Dear Friend,

Do you know that God wants you to be well? He loves you so very much!

"For God loved the world so much that He gave His one and only Son, so that everyone who believes in Him will not perish but have eternal life." John 3:16 (NLT)

He wants you to be well in your mind, body, and spirit, caring for your body with proper exercise, diet, and rest.

"Guard your heart above all else, for it determines the course of your life." Prov. 4:23 (NLT)

God also wants you to care for your spirit. He invites you to have a personal relationship with Him through His Son, the Lord Jesus. If you have not met Him, you can do so, now, by accepting Jesus Christ as your Lord and Savior. Pray this prayer:

Dear Father,

I believe that you love me and gave your Son, Jesus Christ, to die for my sins. Lord Jesus, I receive your gift of salvation. I give my life to You and take You as my Lord.

Welcome to the family!

If you don't own a Bible, try to obtain one. It is God's love letter to you. Read it. He will help you to understand it. Talk to Jesus, your new friend, often, and ask Him to lead you to a church where you can learn about Him.

ABOUT THE AUTHOR

Lesa Lawson, ND is an advocate of nutrition-based wellness and all things natural. She gained her love of natural remedies from her parents and maternal grandmother. A practicing naturopathic doctor, Lawson specializes in alternative therapies that help clients regain their digestive health. She is the founder of LawsOnHealth Wellness Center, a haven of healing in Northern Virginia. Dr. Lawson's first work is the thought-provoking, *Six Lies Women Believe About Their Health.*

Lesa Lawson, ND, CHC, AADP

Naturopathic Doctor

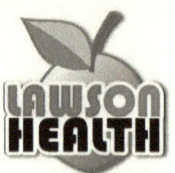

LawsOnHealth Wellness Center

(703) 509-8075

E-mail: Lawsonhealth@gmail.com

Website: Lawsonhealthwellness.com

BOOKS BY DR. LAWSON

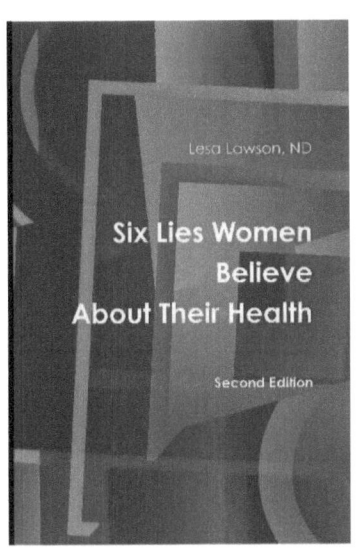

Six Lies Women Believe
About Their Health
Second Edition

Order: http://bitly.com/1sJI7FS
or on Amazon.com

Consultations:

Skype

Phone

Office

Contact Dr. Lawson for schedule and fees:

lawsonhealthwellness.com (website)

lawsonhealth@gmail.com (e-mail)

Order Products

Nature's Sunshine Products
(supplements, herbs, essential oils):
https://www.naturessunshine.com/us/
Sponsor ID#: 3384980

Cherish (Sanitary Pads)
lawsonhealth.nspirenetwork.com or
lawsonhealth@gmail.com

dōTERRA®: *Essential Oils*:
http://mydoterra.com/lesalawson
ID#: 1175848

Kangen Water Machines *(Alkaline Water)*:
www.enagic.com
Distributor ID: #6157558

Air Purification Machines and Laundry Pure
(Clean Clothes without Detergent or Hot Water)
www.vollara.com
Distributor ID: 826463

www.ingramcontent.com/pod-product-compliance
Lightning Source LLC
Chambersburg PA
CBHW050414290526
45786CB00003B/1261